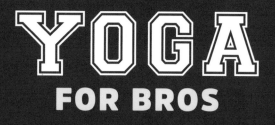

YOGA
FOR BROS

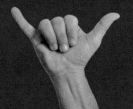

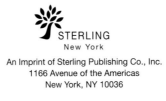

STERLING
New York

An Imprint of Sterling Publishing Co., Inc.
1166 Avenue of the Americas
New York, NY 10036

ISBN 978-1-4549-1957-5

Distributed in Canada by Sterling Publishing, Co., Inc.
c/o Canadian Manda Group, 664 Annette Street
Toronto, Ontario, Canada M6S 2C8
Distributed in the United Kingdom by GMC Distribution Services
Castle Place, 166 High Street, Lewes, East Sussex, England BN7 1XU
Distributed in Australia by Capricorn Link (Australia) Pty. Ltd.
P.O. Box 704, Windsor, NSW 2756, Australia

For information about custom editions, special sales, and premium and corporate purchases, please contact Sterling Special Sales at 800-805-5489 or specialsales@sterlingpublishing.com.

Manufactured in Canada

2 4 6 8 10 9 7 5 3 1

www.sterlingpublishing.com

Photo Credits:
© Depositphotos (can, cup, football, game controller); © iStock (cap, flag, hand gesture)

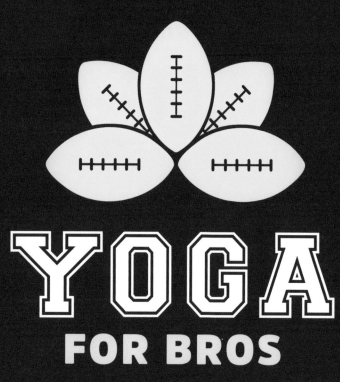

YOGA

FOR BROS

YOUR GUIDE TO MANLY MINDFULNESS

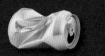

HANNAH ROTHSTEIN

STERLING
New York

A NOTE FROM THE FOUNDER OF YOGA FOR BROS

When I arrived at college, I was lost. Yes, it's true. I, Brogi Brent, didn't know what the hell I was doing. I choked when chugging beers. I was a fail-o at Halo. I couldn't even get chicks into bed. How would I ever get into a frat?

I wandered the campus in shame until the fateful day I stumbled across—or, really, stumbled *over* since I was crunked—the bro who would become my guru.

"I sense you need guidance, young bro," my guru said to me.

"Whaaaaaa?" I replied.

Then, overwhelmed by his extrasensory dudeception and the two measly shots of vodka I'd managed to gulp down, I passed out cold.

When I awoke, I was lying on the floor of an unknown room. Posters of half-naked babes covered the walls, and the space was filled with more weed smoke than furniture. My guru was perched atop a keg, smoking a blunt, doing bicep curls with massive weights, throwing back Red Bulls®, and playing Madden—all at the same time.

Without a word, he threw a protein shake at me. "Bottoms up. Your training begins today."

Under my guru's tutelage, I devoted myself to becoming one with the ways of the bro. I studied hard. Like really fucking hard. Like harder than dweebs do for classes. Then one day, I showed up for my training only to find my guru was nowhere in sight. He had gone off to Colorado in search of the secret to Coors Light®. I shrugged. I wasn't upset. Didn't fucking need him anyway; I was already tapped into the essence of the broniverse.

I knew I couldn't keep the lessons I'd learned to myself. I had to share them with others. How else would they know I was the ultimate fucking bro? This goal in mind, I began to formulate Yoga for Bros.

The creation of the asanas (aka poses) that make up Yoga for Bros came easily to me. I just had to channel the energy of the broniverse every time I did something difficult. Not that anything is hard for me. *Obviously.* Take Lap Dance Chair, for example. That was created when I went to a strip club and there

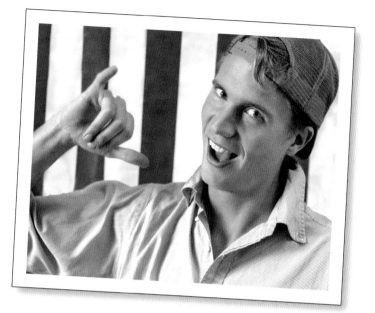

was nowhere to sit. No chair? No problem. I squatted back and raised my arms so as to become a chair myself. And I got five lap dances. In a row. For free. Then, there's Reverse Weekend Warrior. That came to me at a Kappa Sigma party. I'd taken twelve shots and couldn't drink anymore. But then, I found my arm extending and knee bending into a lunge form that let me take more shots than any bro had even seen. EVER.

Now, five years later, I'm the most awesome super senior in the United States of America. I can take thirty-nine shots in one sitting. I can throw a football two miles. I can lift the weight of seventeen cars and get any babe I want just by flexing my left pec. And it's all thanks to Yoga for Bros.

Yoga for Bros lead me down the path to menlightenment. It changed my life . . . and it can change your lame one, too.

Broi Brent

Founder of Yoga for Bros

HOW TO USE THIS BOOK

With a lifestyle of pounding beers, impressing chicks, and getting yoked, there's no one that needs to bliss out more than bros. Happily, Yoga for Bros is here to help the brotastic brethren reach all new levels of zen for men.

This book is structured around the four key facets of the bro being: sports and fitness, partying, girls, and lifestyle. It will give you guidelines for your practice, introduce you to the most pivotal poses, and help you integrate its teachings into your life at large.

So grab a mat, settle into Manchild's pose (pages 12 and 13), and prepare to channel the mantra of Yoga for Bros: Breathe in, bro out.

GUIDELINES FOR YOUR PRACTICE

Clothing

Wear clothing that makes you feel good about how you look, as others are always judging you. We recommended loose-fitting clothes; they allow for ample movement. Tight, spandex garments should be avoided; you should never give anyone reason to question your masculinity.

Time of Day

Although Yoga for Bros can be practiced at any time, poses are often most effective when your proximity to babes and beers is at its peak.

Discomfort

Yoga for Bros is about listening to your body. If a pose causes you pain, consider what your body is saying, then fucking man up.

Environment

Yoga for Bros can be done anywhere. That is the beauty of the practice. But not all settings create an equally satisfying ambiance for Yoga for Bros. Yoga for Bros is best practiced at the following places:

BACKYARD BARBECUES

BENEFIT: The energizing incense of grilled steak ignites the musculature.

THE STADIUM OR GYM

BENEFIT: Easily channel the strength of brogis past, present, and future.

THE CLUB

BENEFIT: The soothing sounds of EDM enhance focus.

THE FRAT HOUSE

BENEFIT: The presence of your fellow bros helps you become one with collective energy of the broniverse.

THE BEACH

BENEFIT: A maximal number of chicks in front of whom you can assert your manliness.

DIVE BARS

BENEFIT: Omnipresent beer will make you more limber.

Breathing Techniques

BREWJJAYI BREATH

This basic breath pattern is employed in many forms of Yoga for Bros. Inhale your favorite brew over the count of five seconds. Hold your breath for five additional seconds. Then, keeping the back of your throat constricted for maximal volume and sound quality, exhale a deep, resonant burp.

SNOTTY SNODHAN BREATH

Place your right index and middle fingers on your forehead. With your thumb resting on one nostril and your little finger on the other, use your thumb to close one nostril. Breathe in slowly, and exhale a massive snot rocket at a nearby bro. Laugh hysterically. Switch nostrils, and repeat.

Props

Some people may tell you that using props is for the weak, but if you've ever tried to get ripped without weights or sliced the shit out of something without a samurai sword, you'll know those people are morons. Props help bros of all experience levels most deeply receive the benefits of their practice. We know some day you'll be able to grill a burger with your bare hands, but until then, props like those below are highly recommended.

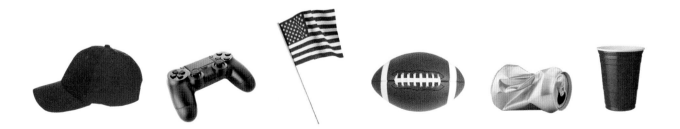

VIDEO GAMEKASANA

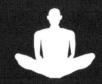

Sit in front of large screen with the bottoms of

your feet touching and your knees bent. Turn on

console and pick up controller. Inhale. Exhale.

Show those motherfuckers who's boss.

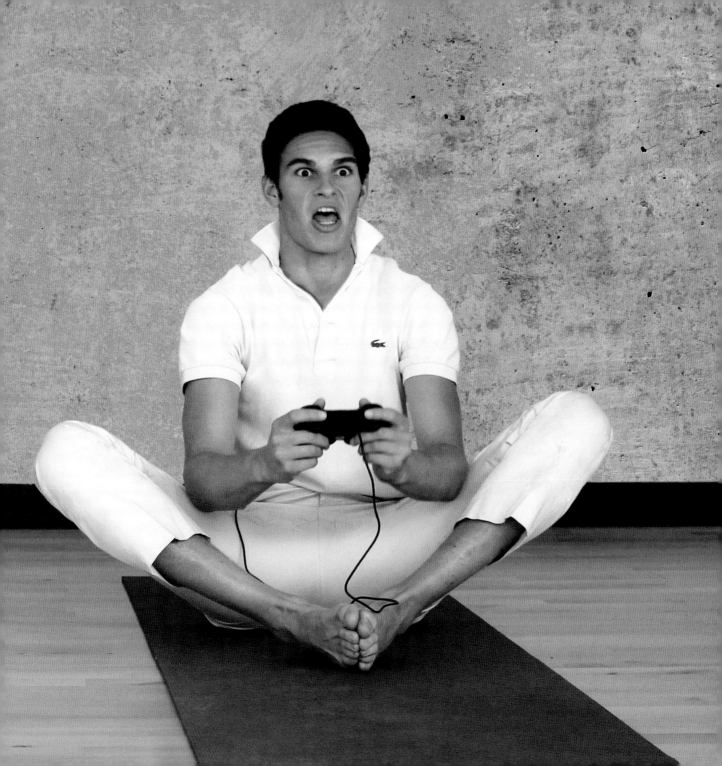

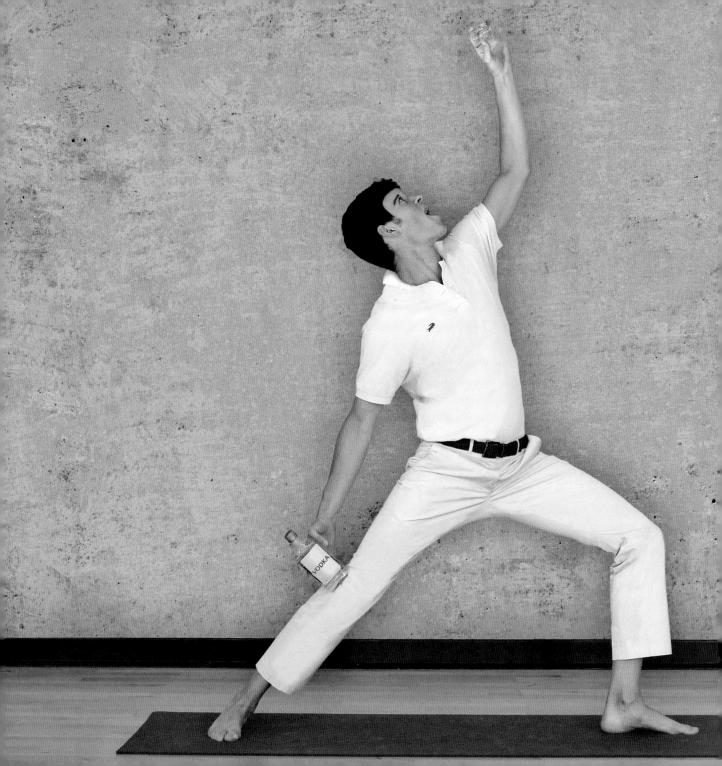

REVERSE WEEKEND WARRIOR

From Linebacker II pose (pages 20 and 21), drop football and grab shot glass. Keeping front knee bent, reach your back arm toward your ankle, and tilt your head.

Now . . . Shots! Shots! Shots!

MANCHILD'S POSE

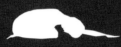

This pose is the foundation of Yoga for Bros. Return to it anytime things become too challenging. With fists clenched, kneel and drape your torso to the ground. If someone asks what you're doing, gesture angrily and reply, "Fuck you, bro. Do you want to take this outside?"

"The greatest challenge in life is discovering who you are. The second greatest is hiding it from everyone else."

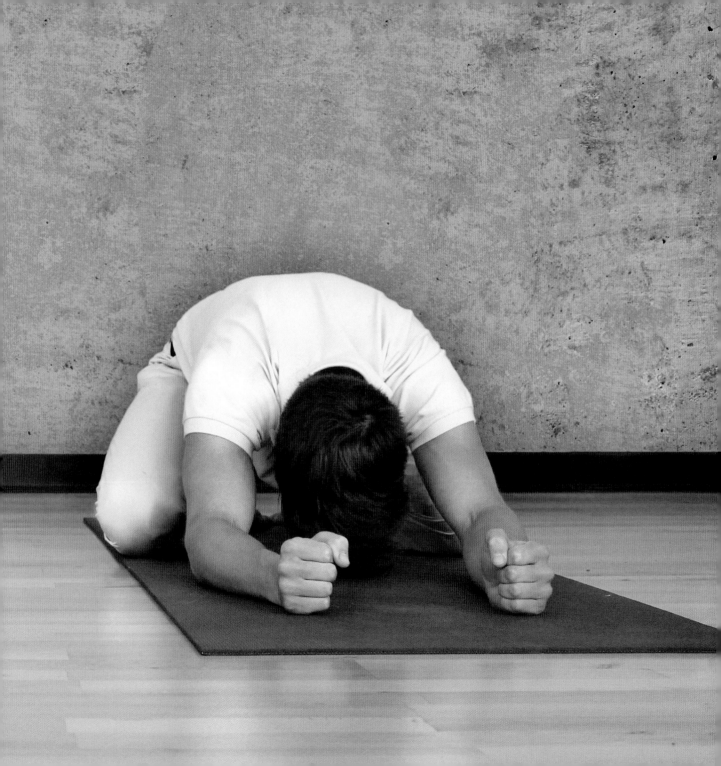

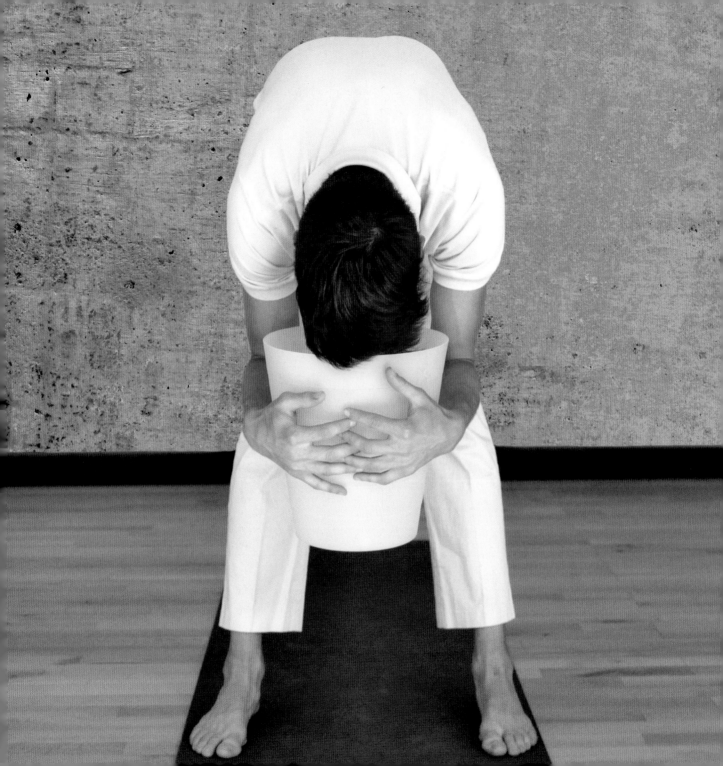

WRECKED DOLL

From drunkenly wobbling on feet, exhale and hinge at hips. Let torso and head hang heavy. Cradle trash can with elbows, and align head with inside of trash can. Puke until you feel release.

KEGSTAND

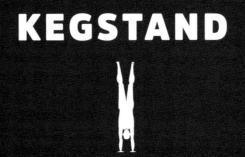

This pose strengthens your arms and brotastic reputation. Place your hands on either side of keg and kick one leg up, followed by the other. Inhale epic amounts of beer.

NOTE: *Though advanced brogis may attempt this pose alone, it is highly recommended that you get an assist for this pose.*

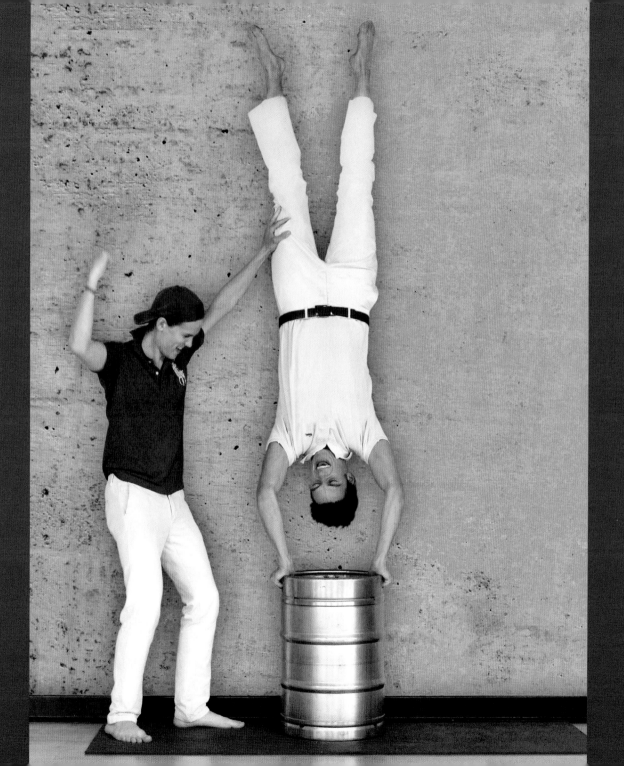

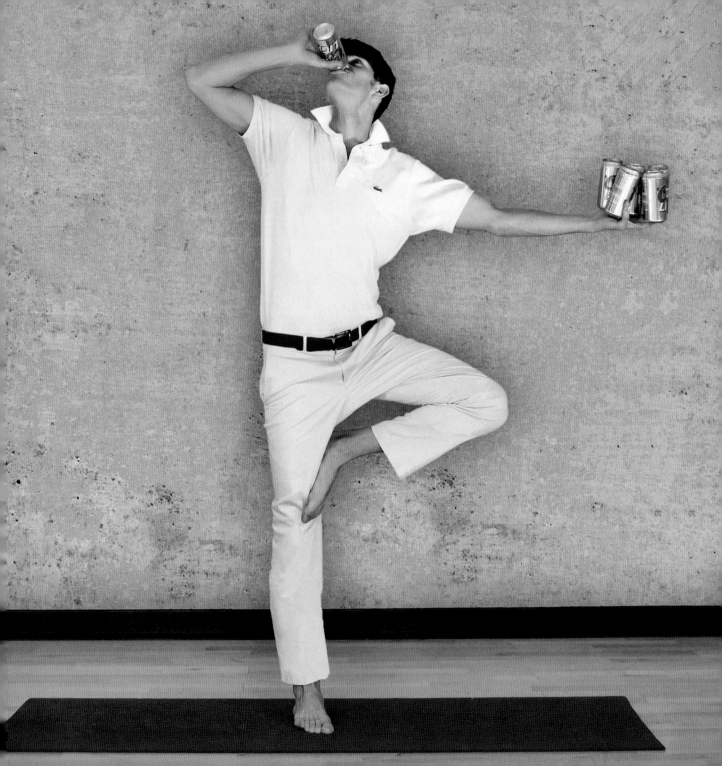

SHOTGUNASANA

Stand tall on one leg with a six-pack in one hand
and your free foot resting on your inner thigh.
Puncture a beer, then pound the shit out of it.

*"By our stumbling, the world
is perfected. Drink up."*

LINEBACKER II

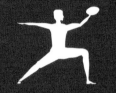

Face the side wall, and bend

your front knee. Hold a football

in your front hand and raise your

arms. Stand at the ready. When

you see a passing freshman,

chuck the football at him with

your Peyton Manning-like skill.

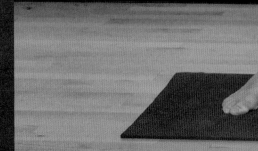

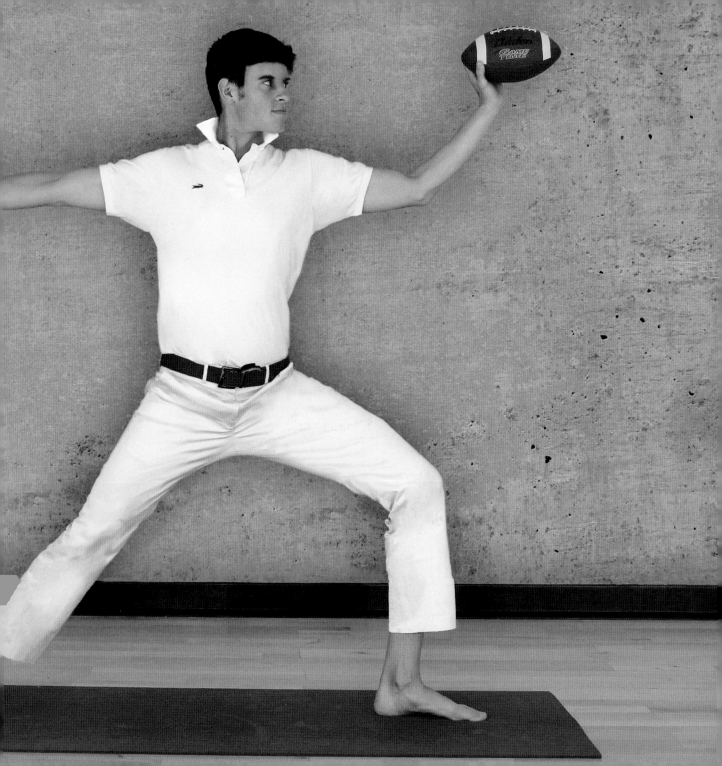

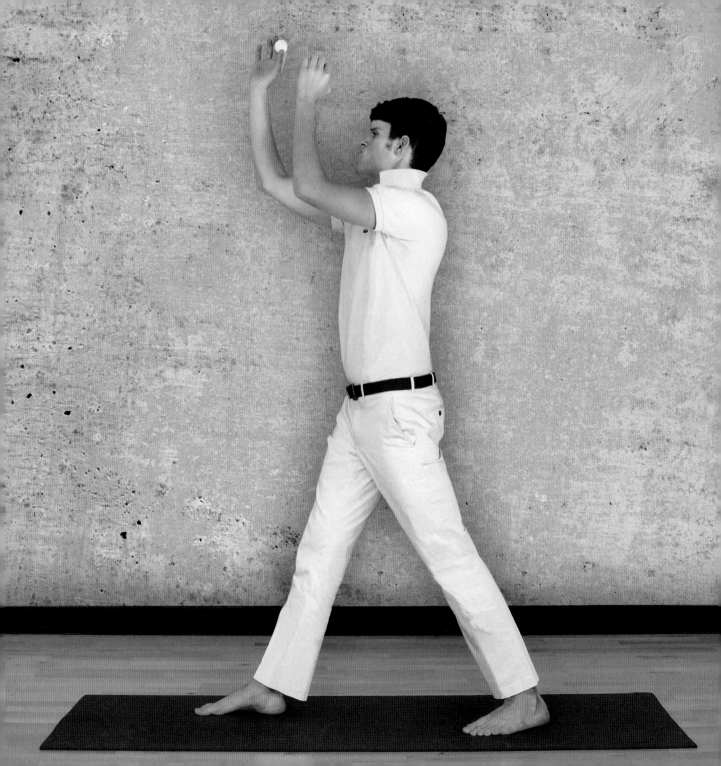

BEER PONG LUNGE

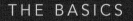

Pick up a Ping-Pong® ball, and step one foot forward.
Inhale and sweep your arms to the sky. Toss the ball and
watch it land in your competitor's cup. Whoop loudly,
and immediately transition into Chest Bump Moon pose.

CHEST BUMP MOON

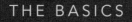

Turn to this pose when the emotions you can't express overwhelm you. It is best done with a partner. Facing your partner, reach your arms to sky, back arched slightly, and bump your chest against his, saying "No homo" as you do.

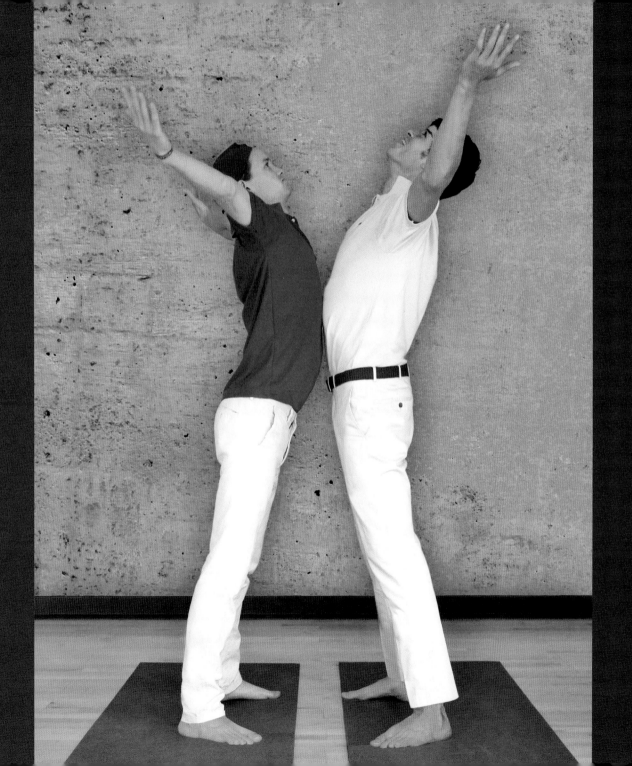

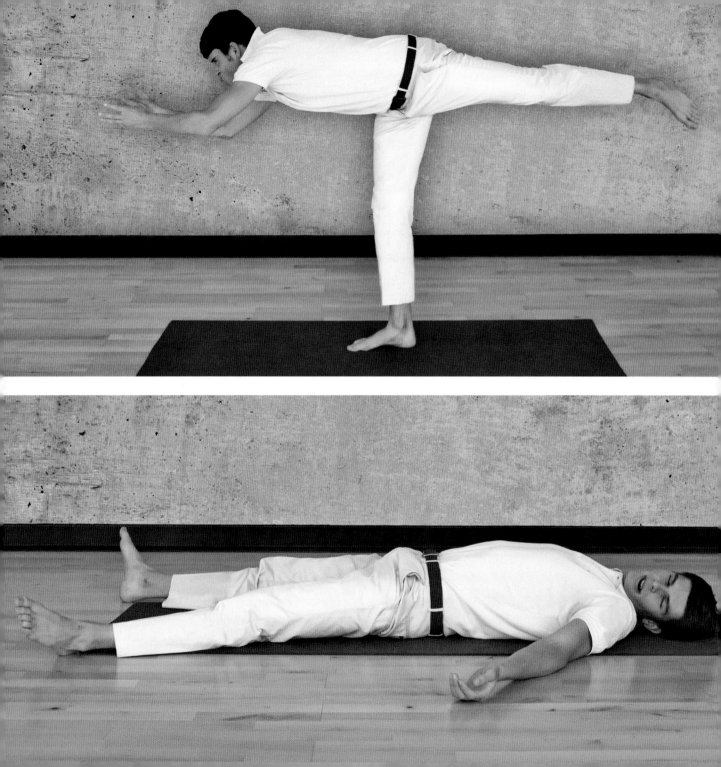

INSENSITIVE BOAR-IOR III

(OPPOSITE TOP)

Balance on one leg and

lean forward with arms

extended. When a hot chick

walks by, make groping

motions with your hands to

display your appreciation

for her womanly form.

SHITFACEASANA

(OPPOSITE BOTTOM)

This is your final pose, your

resting pose. After a night of

partying, fall to the floor with

limbs sprawled wide. If still

cognizant after five minutes,

roll onto your side so you don't

choke on your puke. Breathe

deeply and pass out, bro—

you've done great work today.

SOLO CUP SALUTATIONS

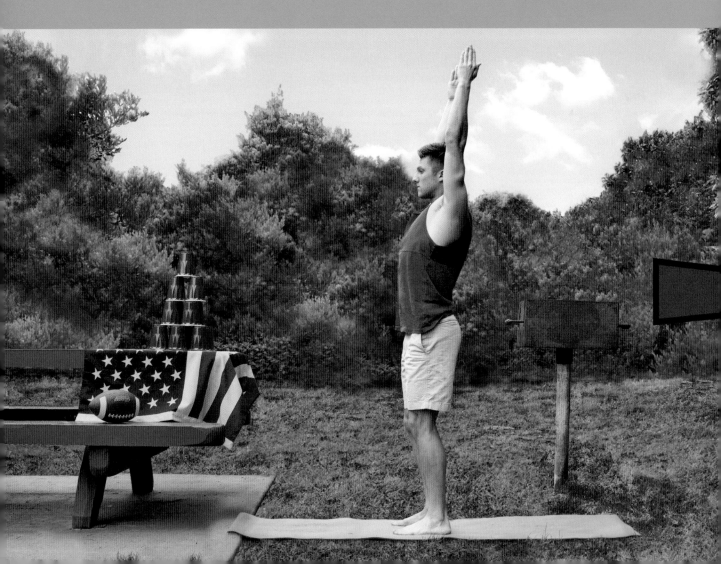

Face a pyramid of solo cups and bring your hands to heart center. Reach up to the sky, then bow forward. Return to standing, then take a cup and party your face off.

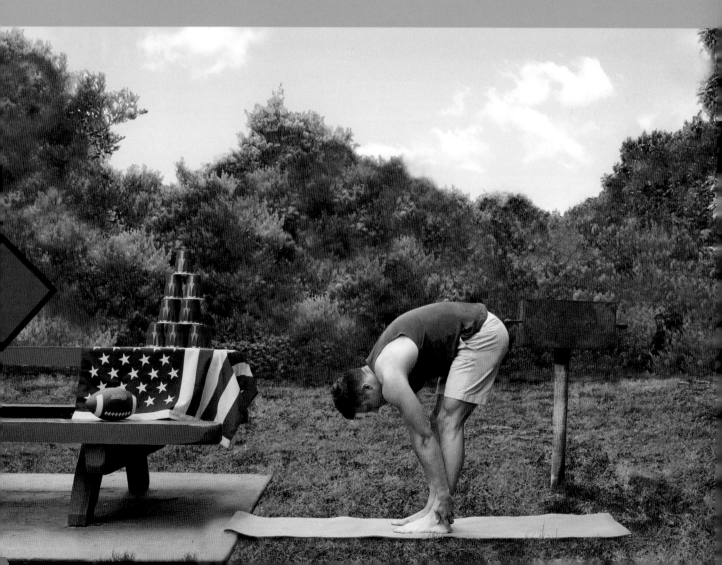

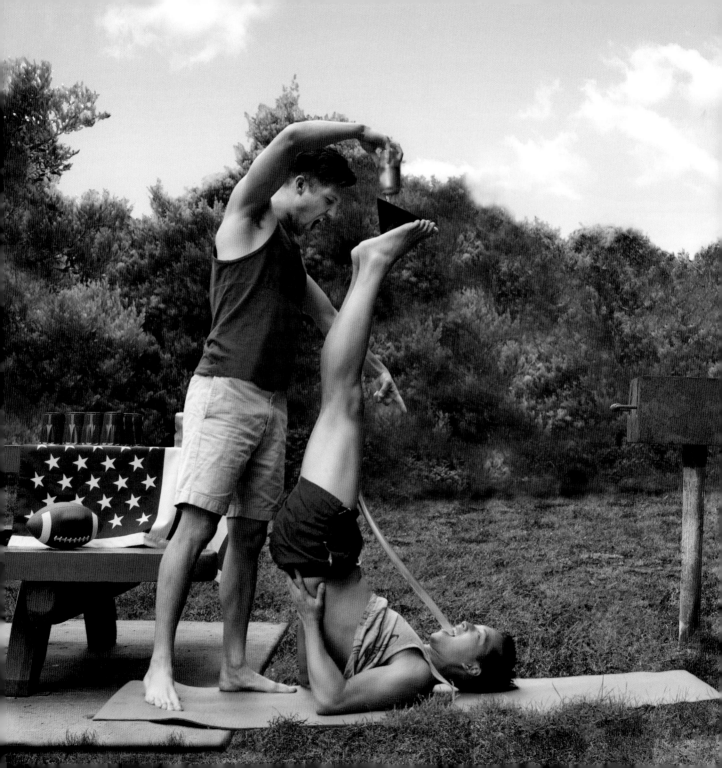

BEER BONGASANA

Turn to this pose whenever you feel sober. Lie down on your back and cradle a beer bong with your feet, raising your legs to the sky. Rest your lower back on your hands and demand that someone pour a brewski into the bong. Soften your belly, then inhale Every. Single. Drop.

"Live in the present, forget the past. Fuck the future, and keep partying."

EXTENDED SLAP-THE-BAG ANGLE

This pose strengthens your level of inebriation. Ask a fellow brogi to hold a bag of wine beside you. Plant your feet wide, inhale, and bend your front knee. On your next exhale, slap that bag and transition into High Belch Lunge (pages 80 and 81).

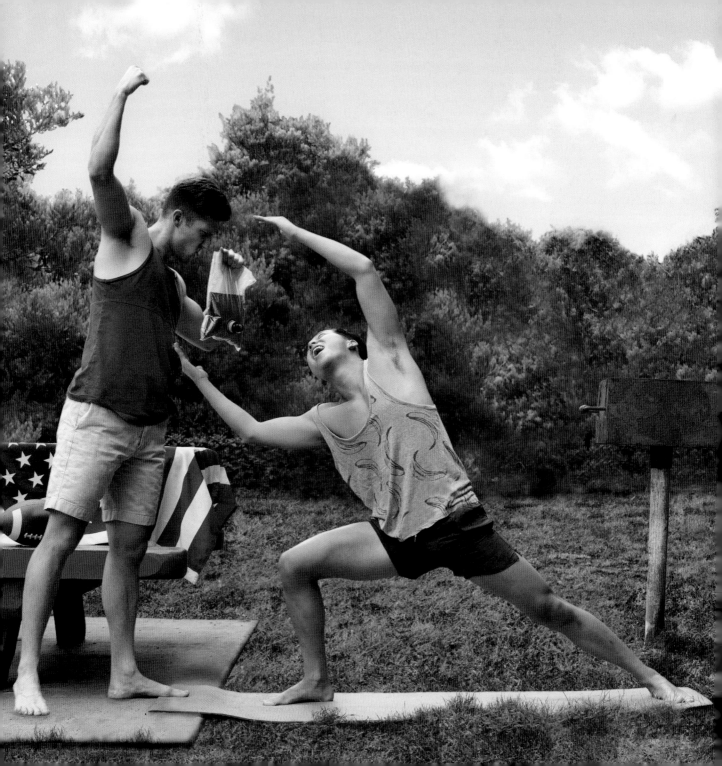

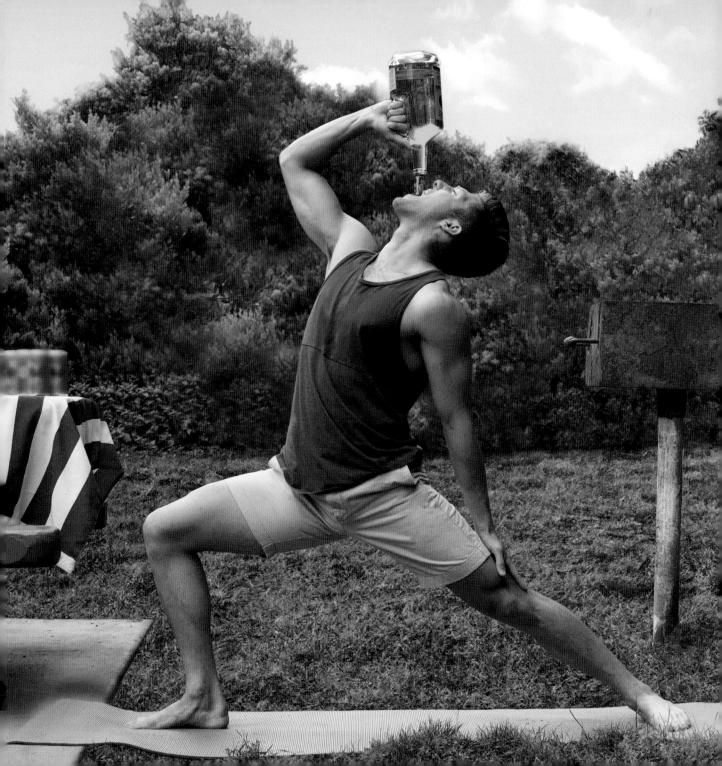

ADVANCED WEEKEND WARRIOR

Some believe you should master Reverse Weekend Warrior before attempting this pose. Those people are pussies. Follow the steps for Reverse Weekend Warrior (pages 10 and 11), using a handle instead of a shotglass. Chug until you reach Shitfaceasana.

CRUSHING CAN LUNGE

From Shotgunasana, step your raised foot to the back of the mat. Place a beer can in your palm, and bend your front knee. On an exhale, crumple the can against your forehead with a loud, manly cry.

"When I let go of what I am, I'm probably stoned out of my mind."

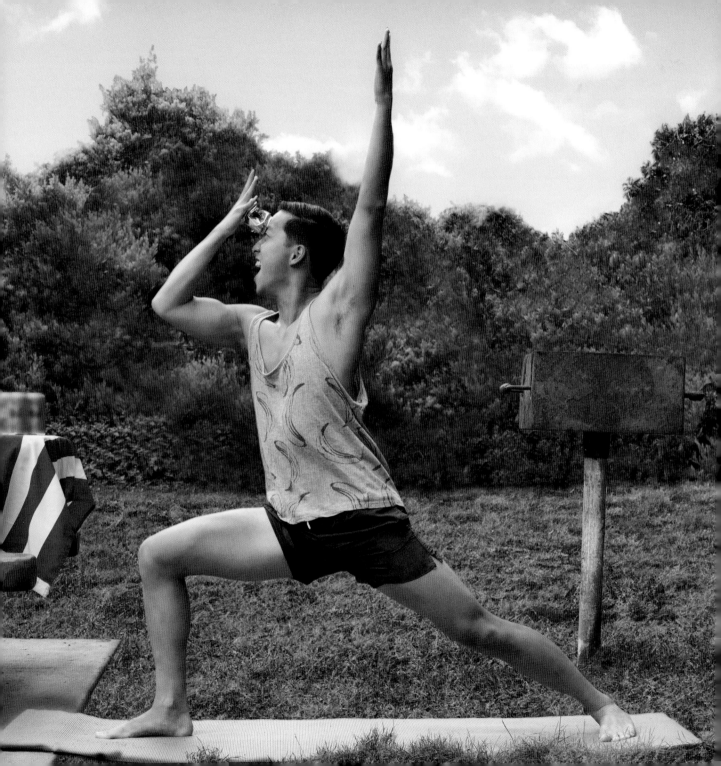

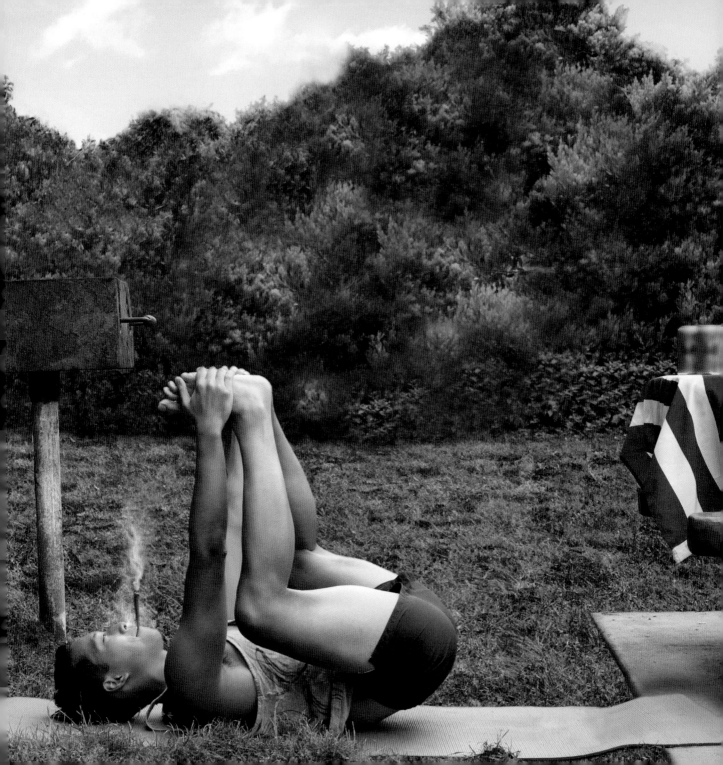

HAPPY BAKEY POSE

With a blunt between your lips, lie down on your back and take your feet to the sky. Catch the outsides of your feet, and inhale deeply for a count of five. Hold your breath, then exhale slowly. Laugh hysterically about nothing, then repeat.

MINI FRIDGE TWIST

Best for relieving nausea, cranial discomfort, and pain caused by shitty life choices, this is one of Yoga for Bros' most restorative poses. Squat low, and bring your hands to heart center. Twist from your hips as you reach to open the fridge. Grab a cold one, and drink until your hangover goes away.

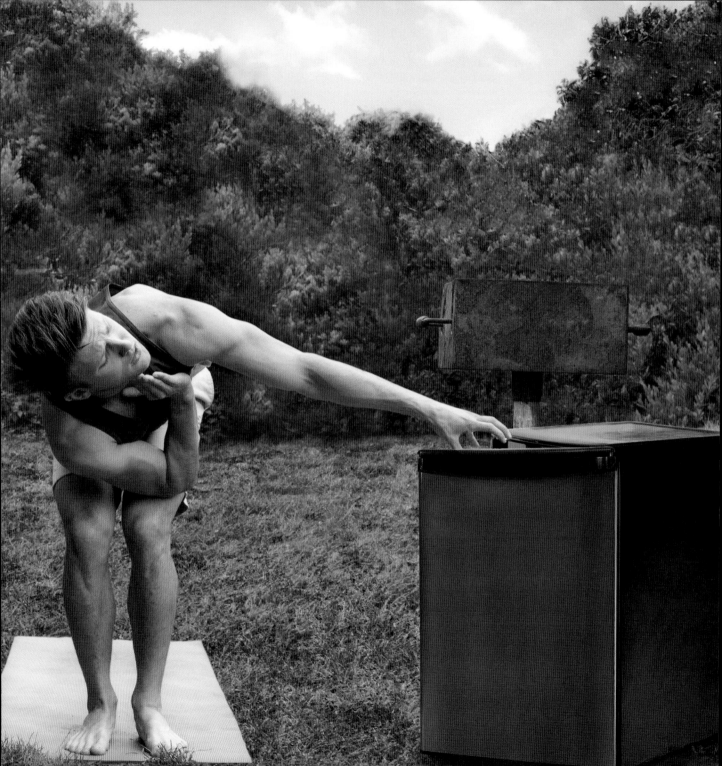

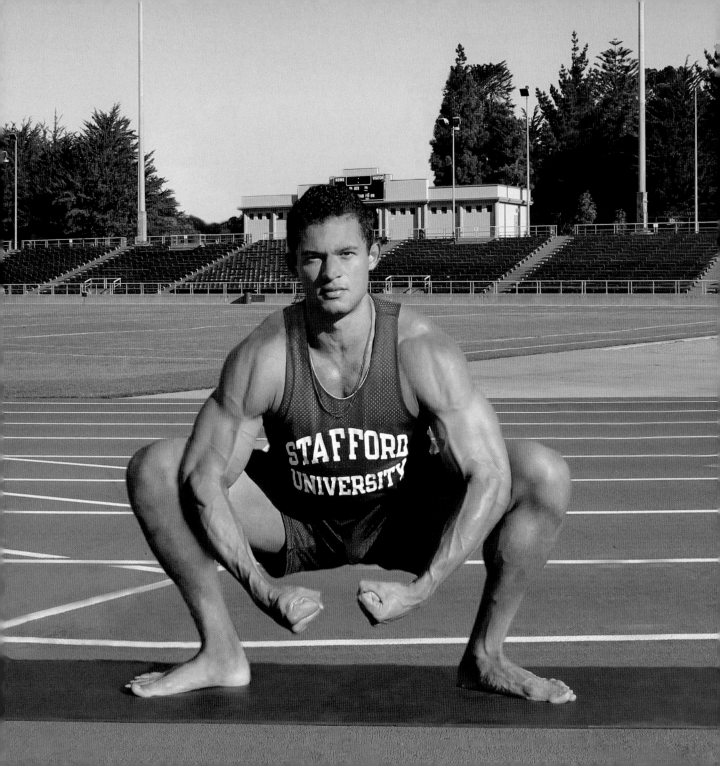

MUSCLASANA

This pose affirms your manliness. Squat deep, and make your hands into fists. Engage your muscles. Flex. More. Until every sinew stands erect. Perfect. You are a fucking god.

LORD-OF-THE-LIFTING POSE

Hold a weight in one hand and raise your opposite foot behind you. Reach back with your free hand, grab your foot, and lean forward. Raise the dumbbell high and yell, "Go big or go home!"

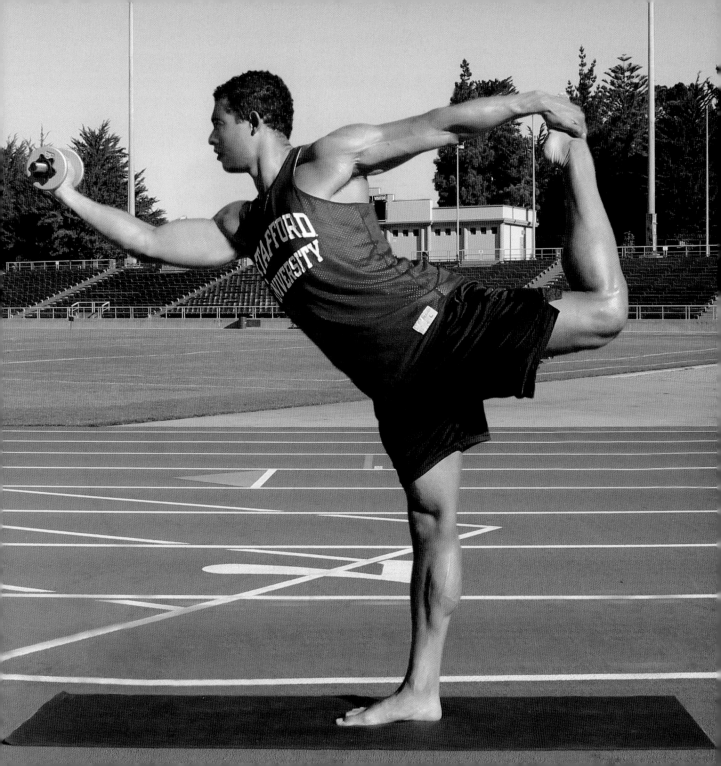

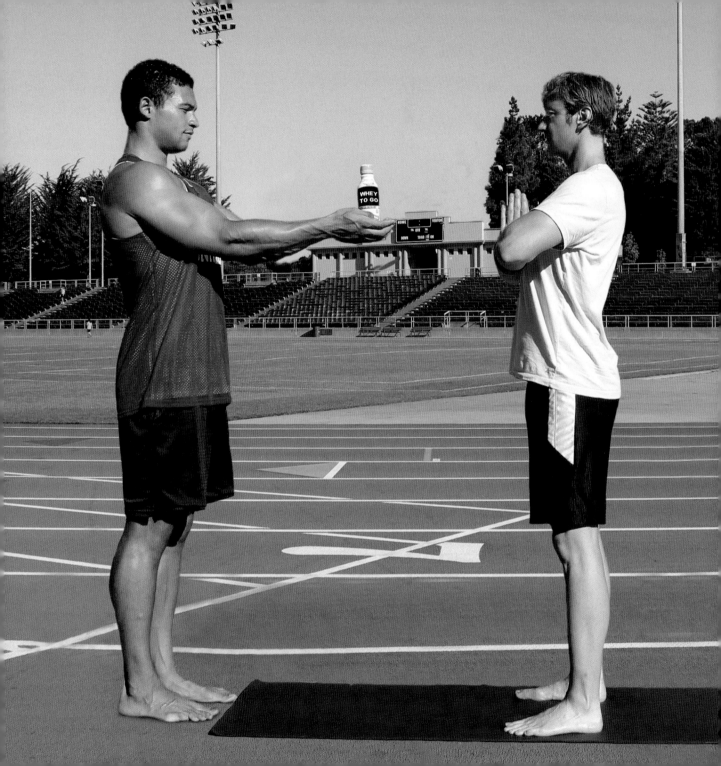

PROTEIN SHAKE SALUTE

Facing your favorite protein shake, stand tall and bring your hands to heart center. Focus your gaze on the miraculous bottle of brotein. Remain in the pose until you feel swole.

TOUCHDOWN TRIANGLE

This pose is best done with a partner.

With letters painted on your chests,

take a wide stance. Place your front

hand on your calf and wait. When

your home team scores, raise your

arm, and shout victoriously.

*"The quieter you become,
the more you hear what
a moron everyone else is."*

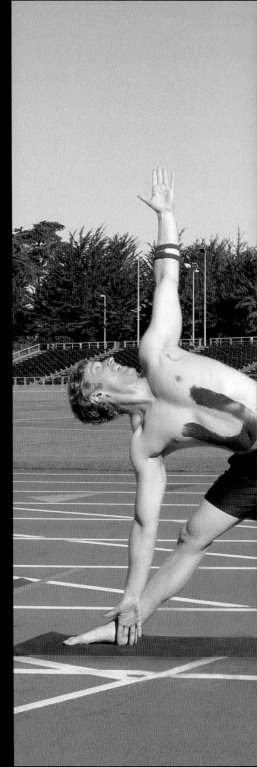

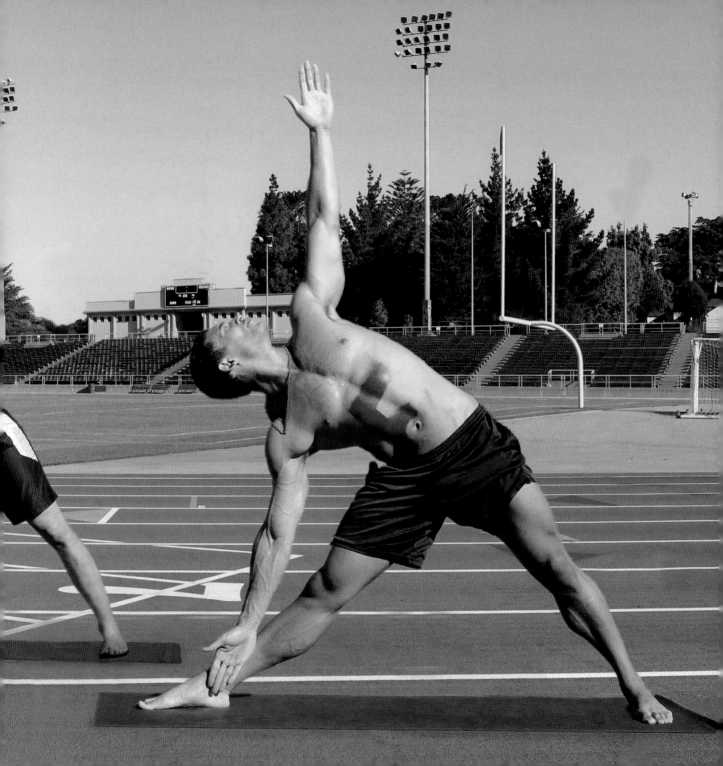

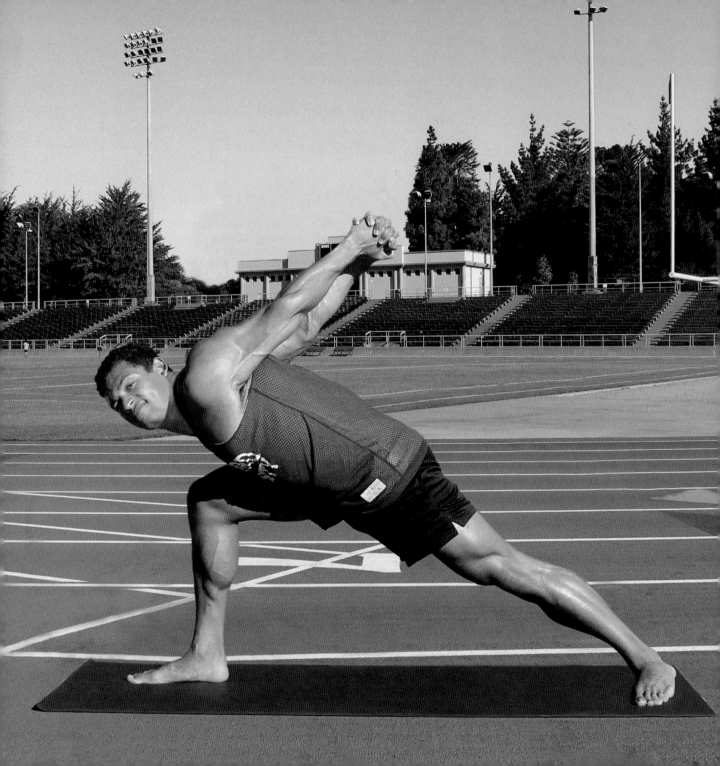

NOT-SO-HUMBLE WARRIOR

Lace your fingers behind your back and step into a lunge. Flex your muscles to show how yoked you are, and fold forward. Looking smug, take a few minutes to meditate on just how awesome you are.

WEIGHT ROOM HERO TWIST

Grab two weights and sit back on your calves. Twist to one side, furrow your brow intently, and lift the weights to 90° angles. Hold the pose until everyone in sight notices your incredible strength.

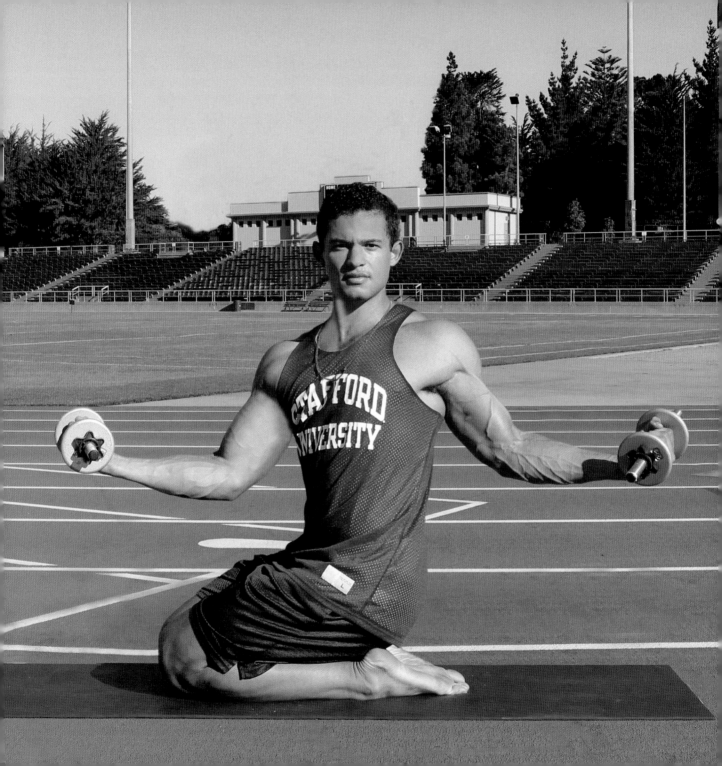

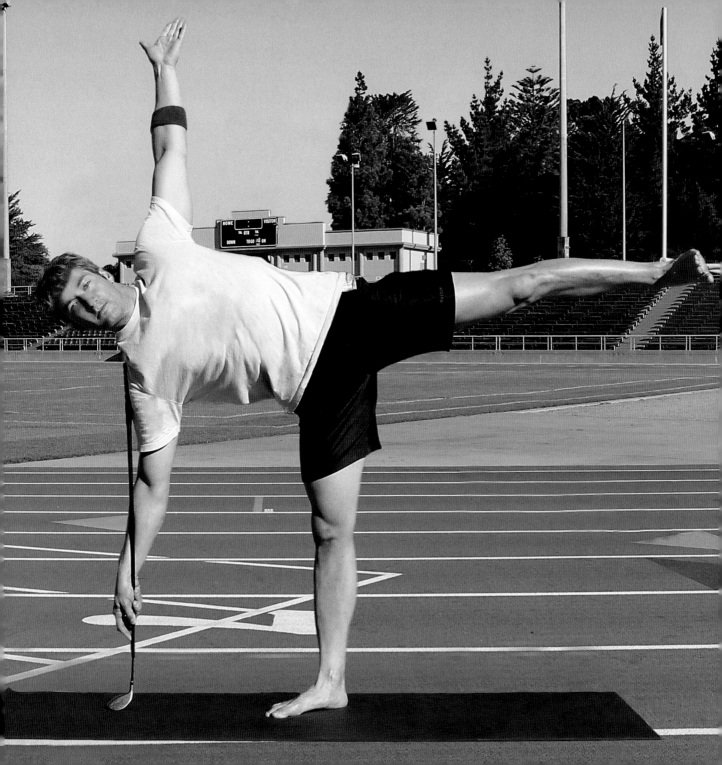

HALF GOLF MOON

Often practiced on the green, this pose improves your ability to score below par. Hold a golf club upright and balance on one foot. Rotate your torso to the sky. Look toward the hole until you've assessed the best way to land a hole in one.

BEER TO BICEP

Often practiced during tailgates and parties, this pose helps connect you to the energy of the broniverse. Stand tall. Balance a beer on your upper arm and flex. Keep the pose for a count of five, then move into Not-So-Humble Warrior.

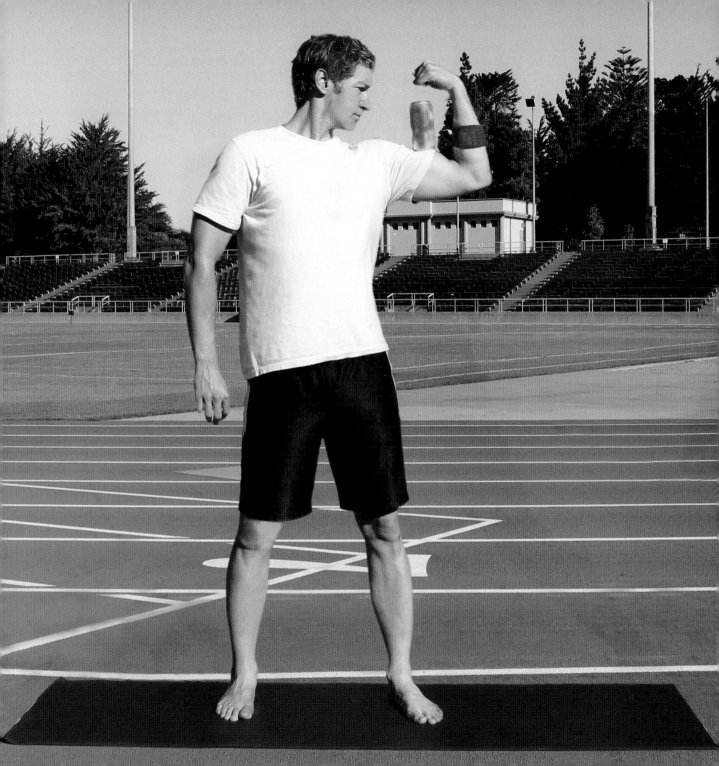

DOWNWARD DOGGIE STYLE

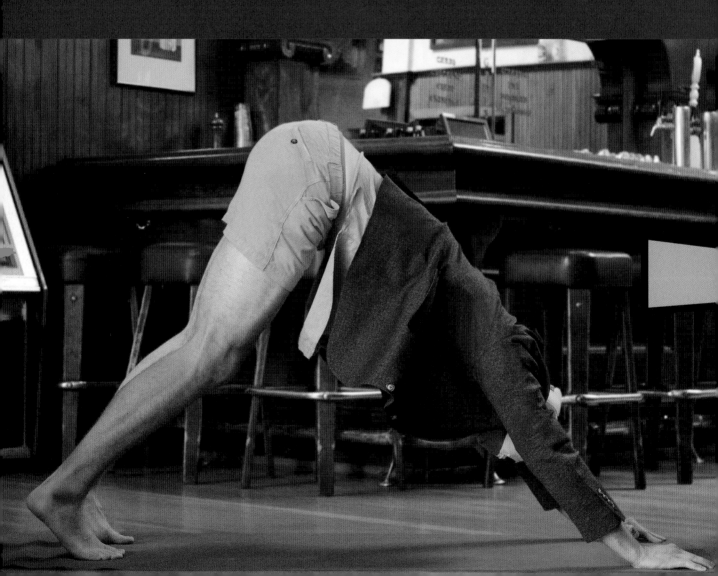

Begin on all fours. Lift your tailbone to form an upside-down V shape.

Inhale. Bend your knees and bring your hips forward with a loud exhale.

Repeat this sequence in quick succession until you feel release.

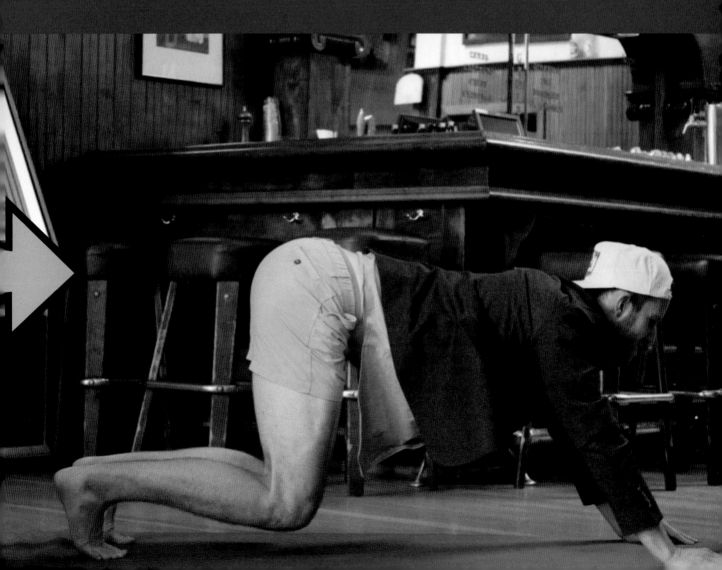

UPWARD LOOKING DOG

This poses increases your libido. When

a girl approaches, lie down on your

belly and push up through your hands.

Raise your eyes to her rear, soften your

gaze, and exhale a loud, "Mmm."

NOTE: *Approach this posture carefully.*
Pushing it too far may result in injury.

"The root of suffering is attachment.
Avoid a serious girlfriend at all costs."

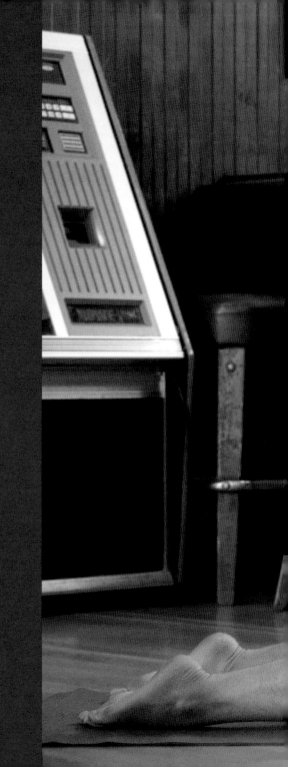

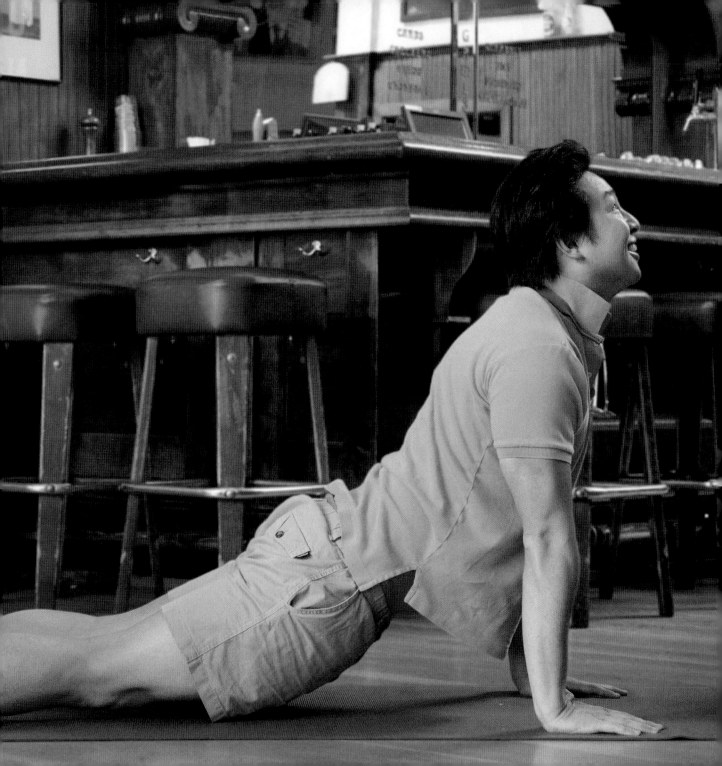

GODDESS PASSANA

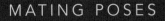

Stand with your feet wide and toes pointed out. Squat low to be out of the line of sight. When a hot girl passes, point and turn your body to follow her movement. If you wish to use an assist, employ binoculars at any time.

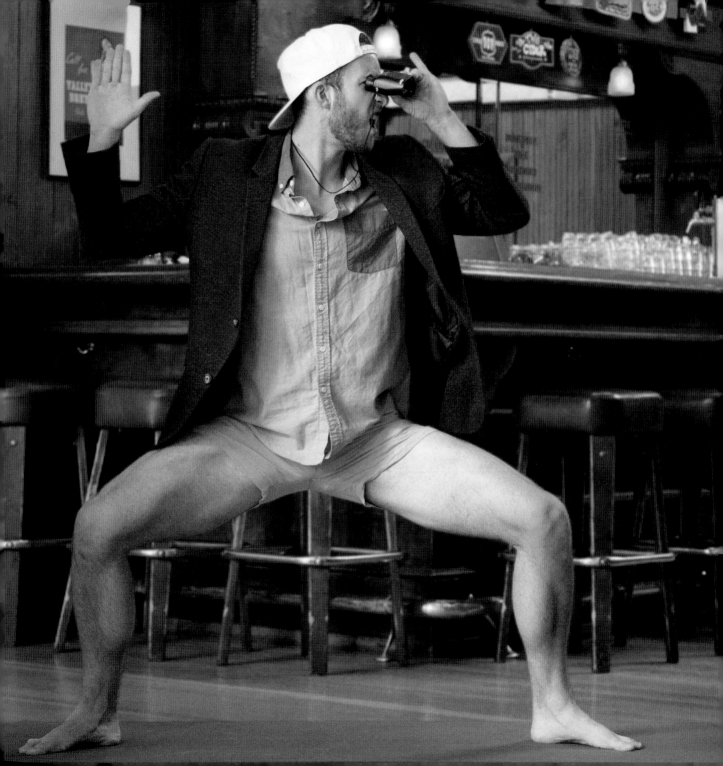

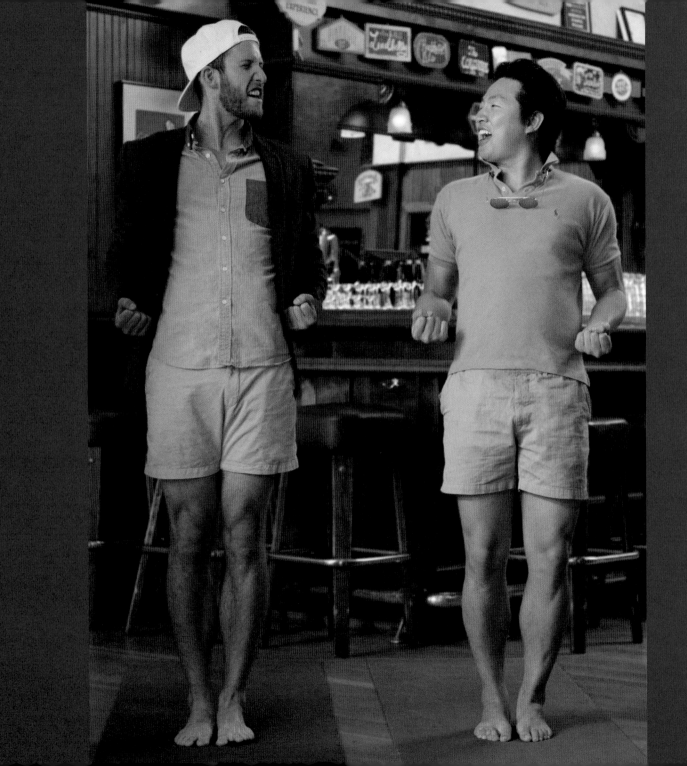

TAPTHATASSANA

Keeping your feet together and hands at your sides, locate the hottest girl in the room. Make eye contact with her and clench your fists. Holding your gaze, move your hips forward and fists back. Repeat until your intentions are clear.

NOTE: *This pose can also be practiced alongside a fellow brogi. Add an exchange of suggestive commentary to help push each other to a new level of lewd.*

BOW BEFORE HOE

This pose displays your

menlightenment. When you

notice a fellow brogi is whipped,

sit down and raise your legs.

Balancing on your tailbone, make

a giant X with your arms. Look at

the offending brogi and exhale

a loud, buzzer-like sound.

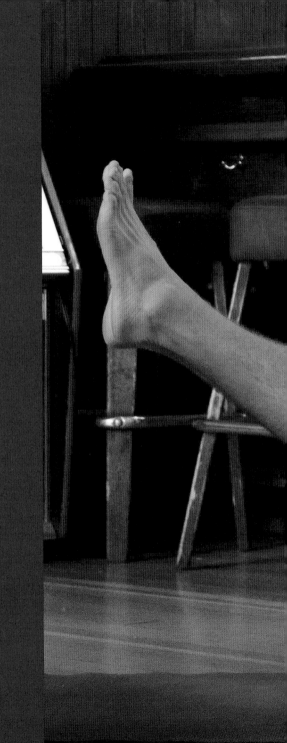

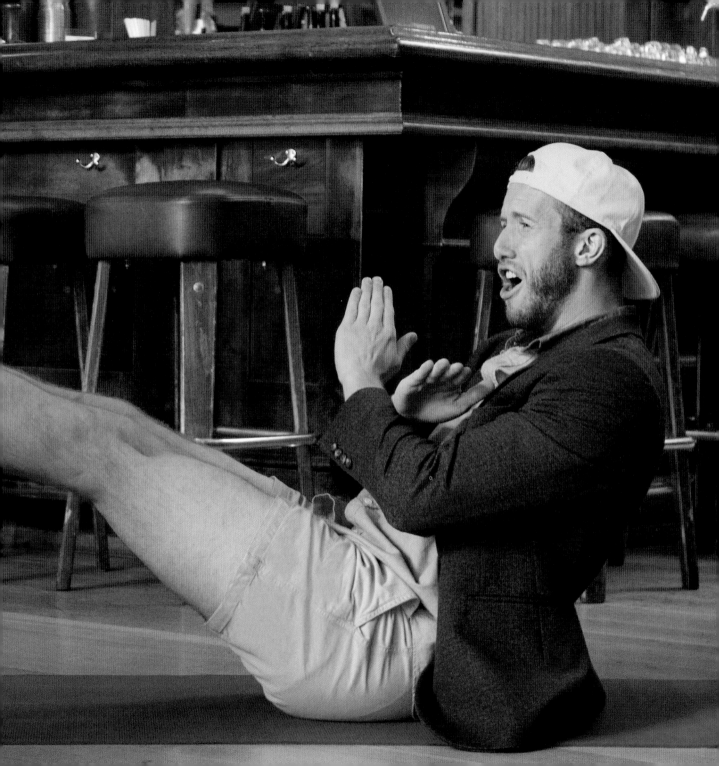

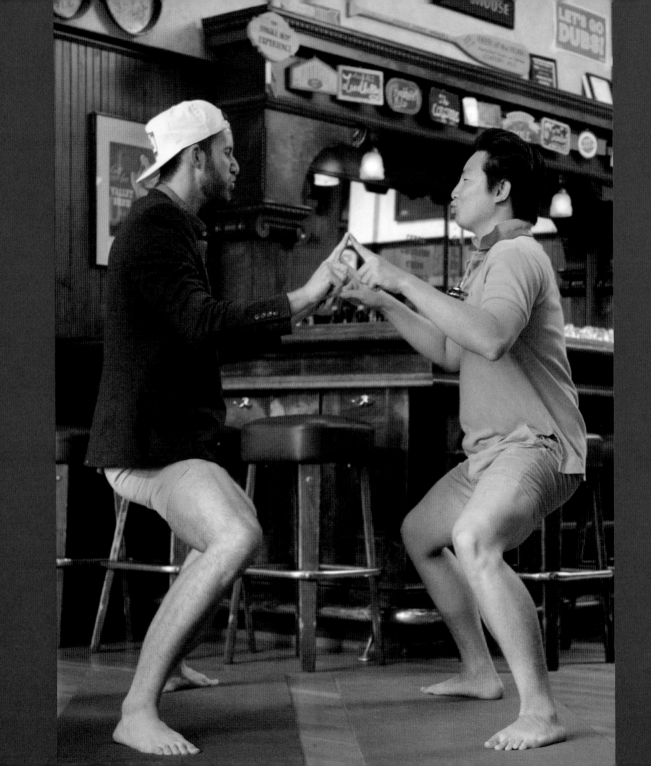

TWIN GODDESS

This pose can be done solo, or with the help of a partner.

Step between two girls. Take a wide stance and squat low.

Bring your pointer fingers together and rotate them back

and forth to express a desire for the girls to make out.

*"Yoga for Bros is
not about self-improvement,
it's about self-abasement."*

LAP DANCE LIGHTNING POSE

A good alternative to Goddess

Passana, this pose flexes your

philandering. With legs together

and a twenty in one hand, squat

low and raise your arms to the sky.

Focus your gaze on a girl. Wave

the twenty, and if it feels good,

move your hips suggestively.

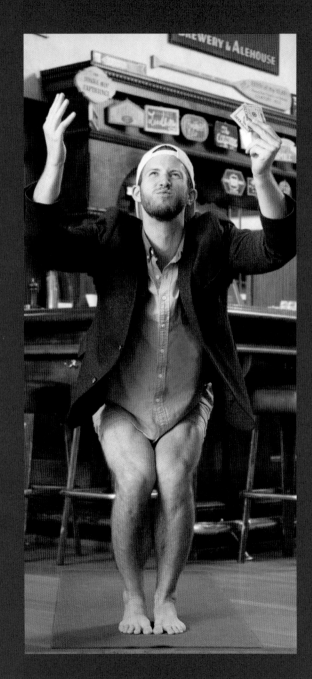

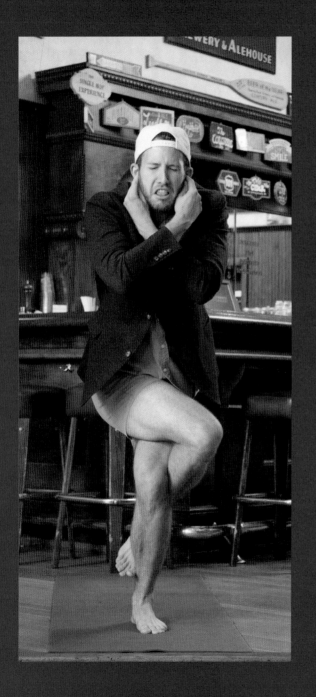

FREE EAGLE OR GIRLAVOIDASANA

This pose often follows

Downward Doggie Style (pages

58 and 59). At the first sign of

a DTR (define the relationship)

talk, stand up and bring one leg

over the other. Cross your arms

at the elbows and place your

fingers in your ears. Scream, "La

la la la la," until the talk stops.

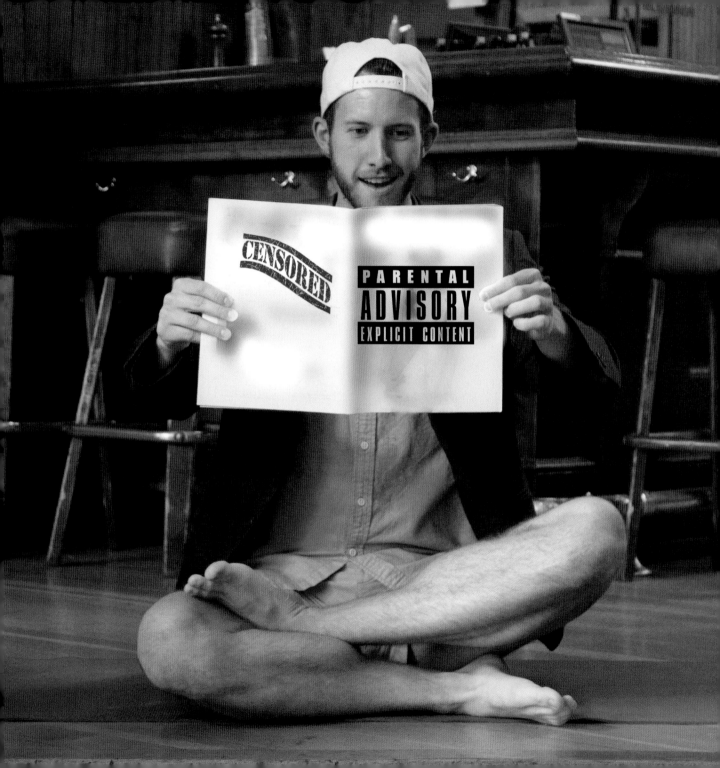

FIRE LOIN POSE

A pornographic magazine is needed to reach the full expression of this pose. Sit down, and stack one calf on top of the other. Open your magazine to a page featuring naked babes and stare until your brain melts.

HALF LORD OF THE LAZYBONES

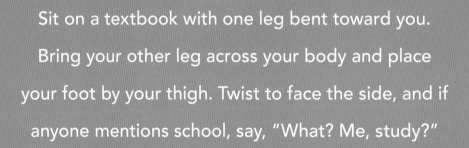

Sit on a textbook with one leg bent toward you. Bring your other leg across your body and place your foot by your thigh. Twist to face the side, and if anyone mentions school, say, "What? Me, study?"

NOTE: *Advanced brogis may wish to use a prop to get deeper into the pose. We recommend a blunt.*

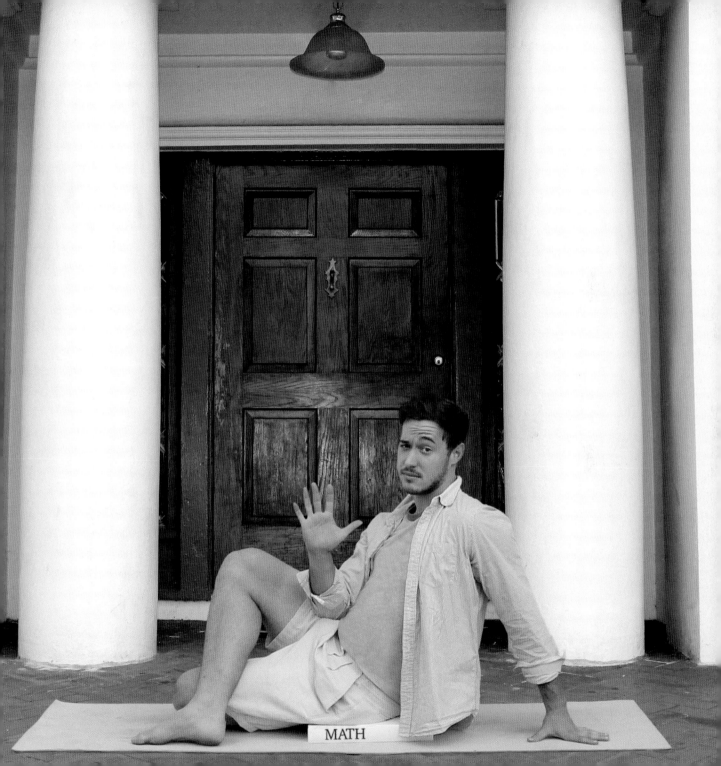

MATH

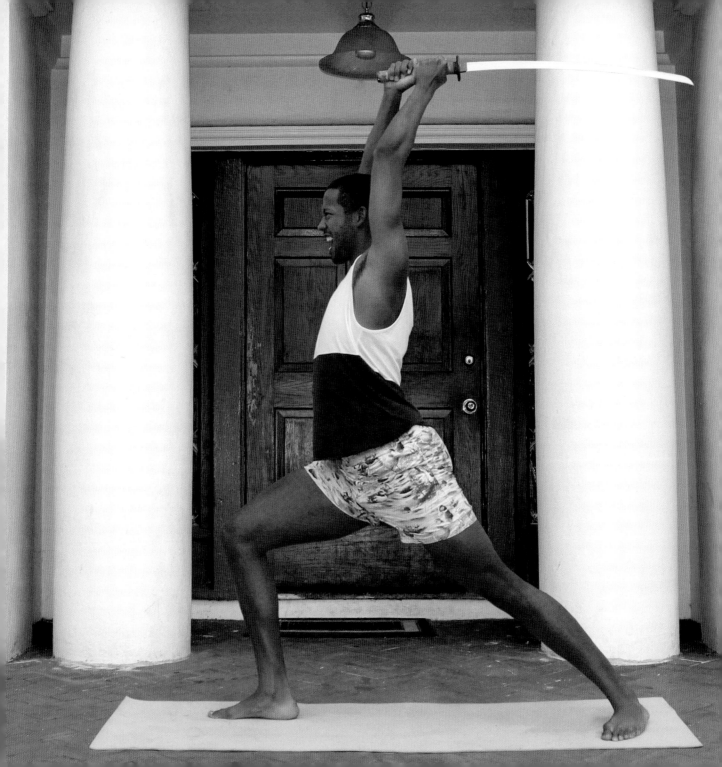

SAMURAI WARRIOR I

From Advanced Weekend Warrior, embrace liquid courage and grab a samurai sword. Keeping your legs wide, face the front and raise the sword. Inhale to steady drunken swaying. Exhale and chop the shit out of a nearby object of your choice.

LOW BELCH LUNGE

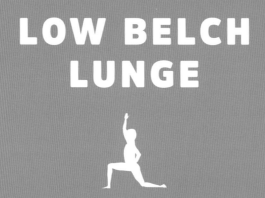

Use this pose to lengthen your signature bump.
Bring one foot to the front and place your back
knee on the ground. Place one hand on your belly
and raise the other one to the sky. When it
feels right, exhale a deep, resonant burp.

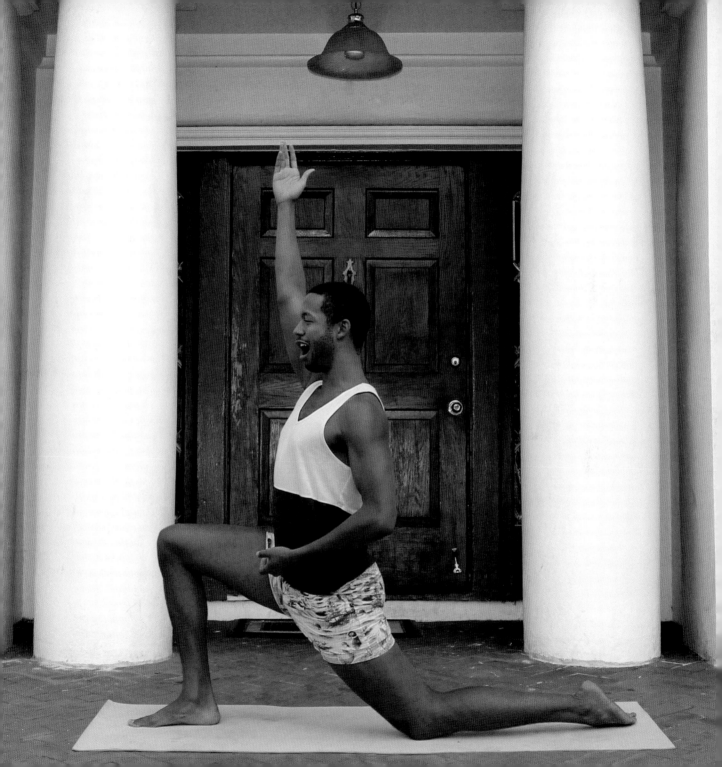

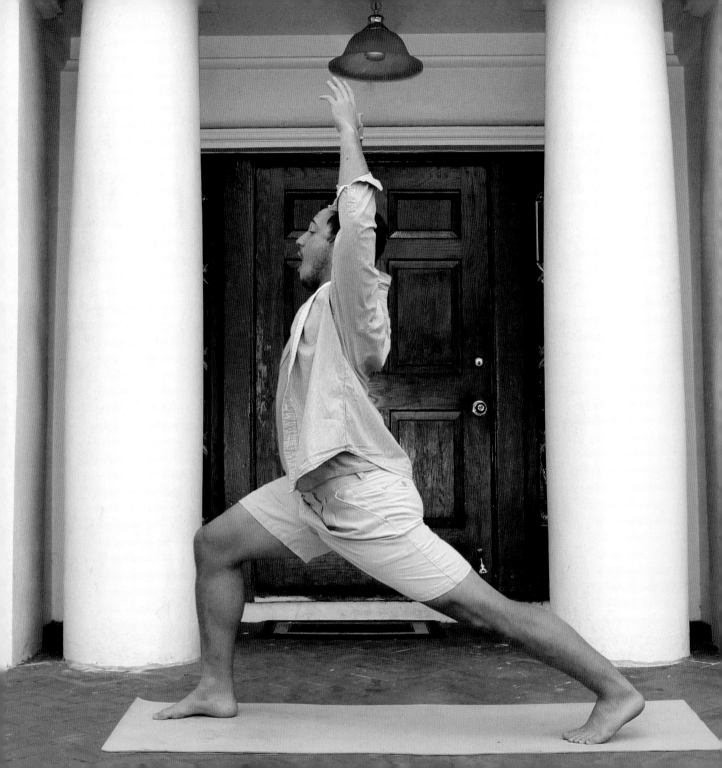

HIGH BELCH LUNGE

From Low Belch Lunge, raise your back knee up and take your fists to the sky. Inhale, then release a burp so loud it shatters every eardrum for miles around. Fratastic, bro. That was a good one.

"Life is about balance—work on your ability to hold a burger, beer, blunt, football, and flag all at the same time."

EXTENDED HAND TO GRILL

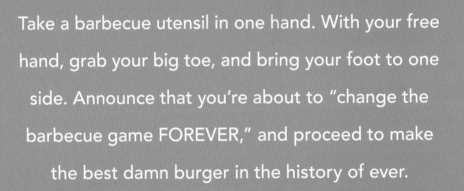

Take a barbecue utensil in one hand. With your free hand, grab your big toe, and bring your foot to one side. Announce that you're about to "change the barbecue game FOREVER," and proceed to make the best damn burger in the history of ever.

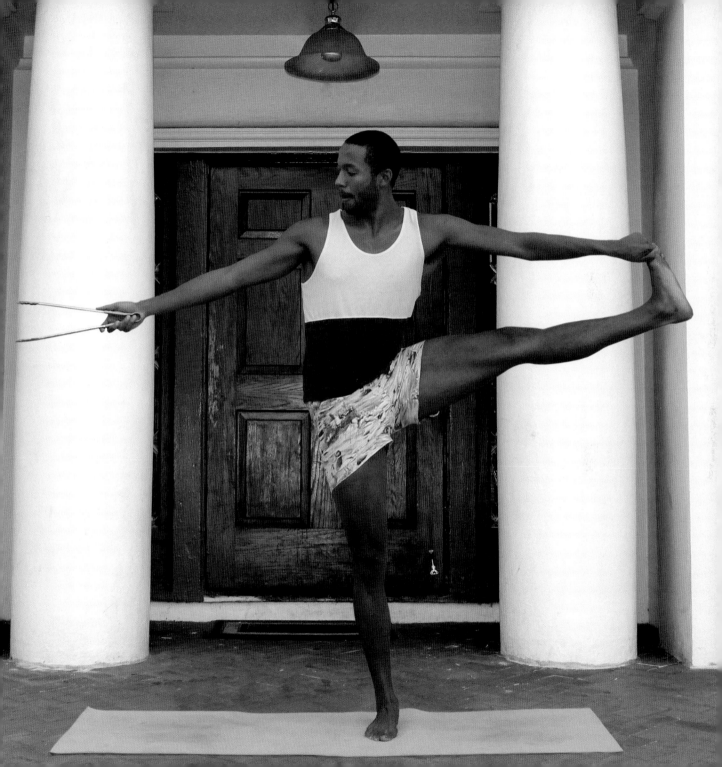

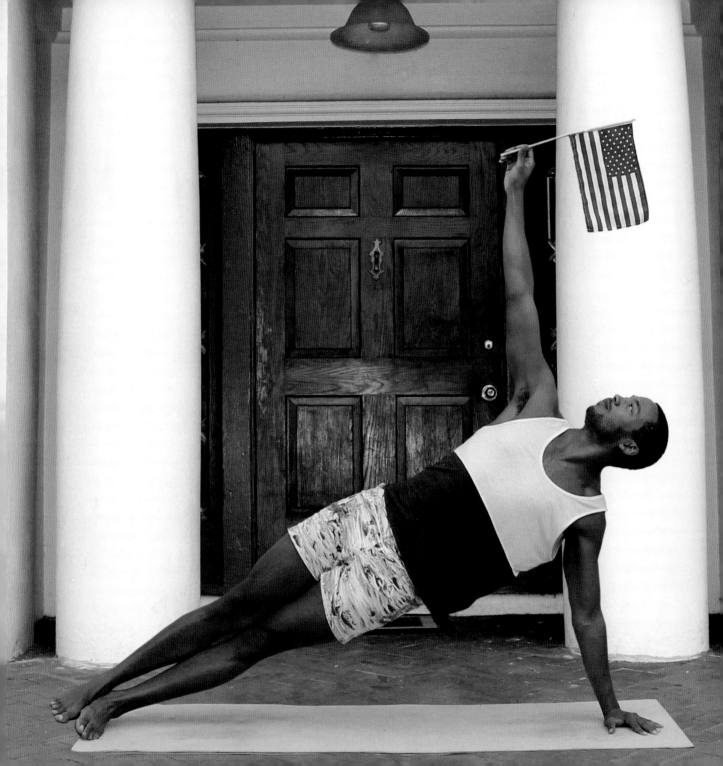

PATRIOTICALLY INCLINED PLANE

When you feel an America boner coming, grab a flag and get into push-up position. Turn to one side as you raise the flag to the sky. Look up and chant the sacred brogi mantra "USA! USA!" as loudly as possible.

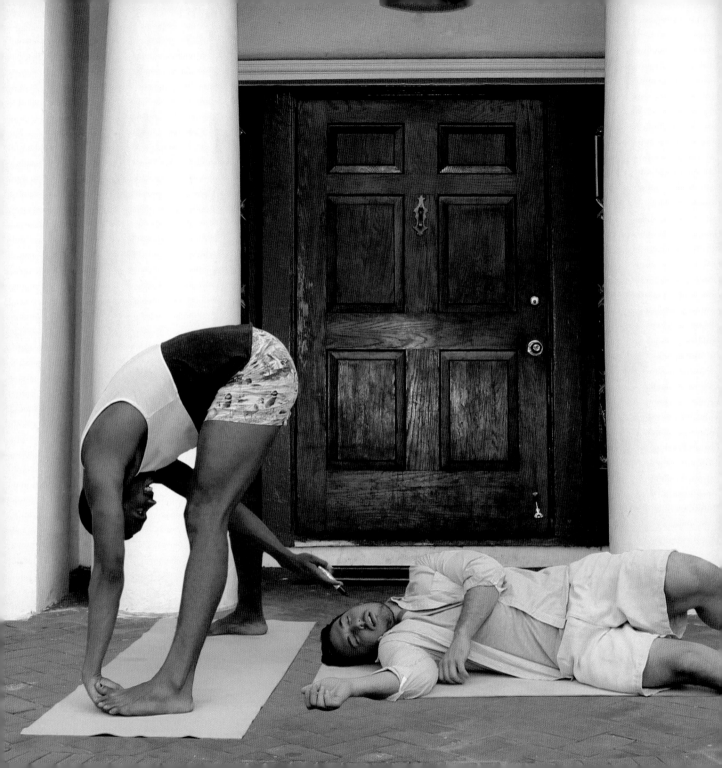

GUERILLA

Also called Sharpie to Face Pose, this stretch requires the presence of a brogi in Shitfaceasana. Stand with feet hip-width apart, grab a permanent marker, and fold forward. Place your free hand under one foot, and use the marker to trace a nice, big dick on your fellow brogi's face.

"Everything you need lies within yourself—and the bottles of beer in your mini fridge."

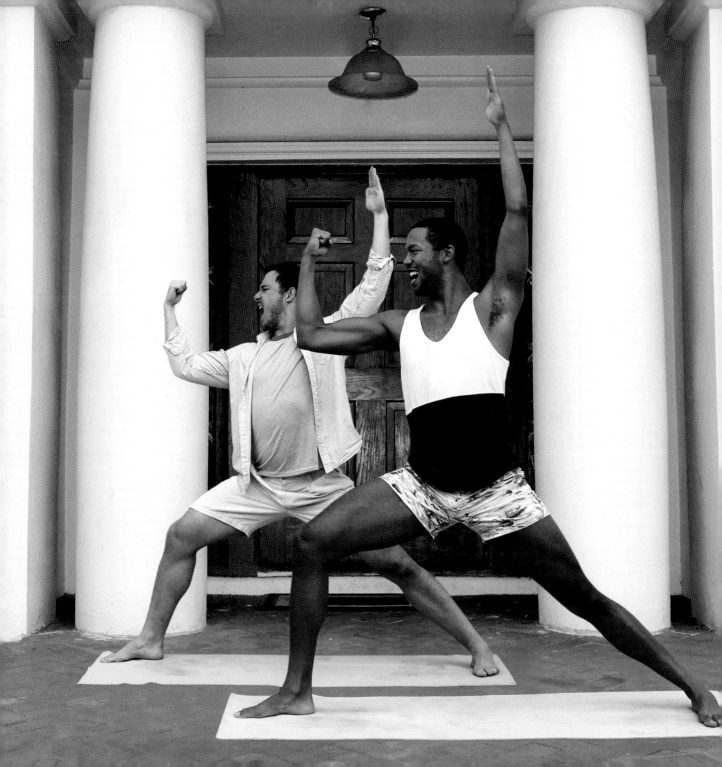

FIST PUMP WARRIOR

Following any accomplishment big or small, step wide and bend your front knee. On an inhale, raise your fist high. On an exhale, lower it with a loud *whoop*. Repeat until all in earshot take note of your success.

WIDE-LEGGED FART BEND

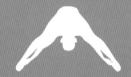

When you feel a fart brewing, stand with your legs wide and soften your torso toward the floor. Grab your big toes, and aim your ass at a fellow brogi. Let one rip and laugh obnoxiously as your fellow brogi crumples under the deathly smell of your flatulence.

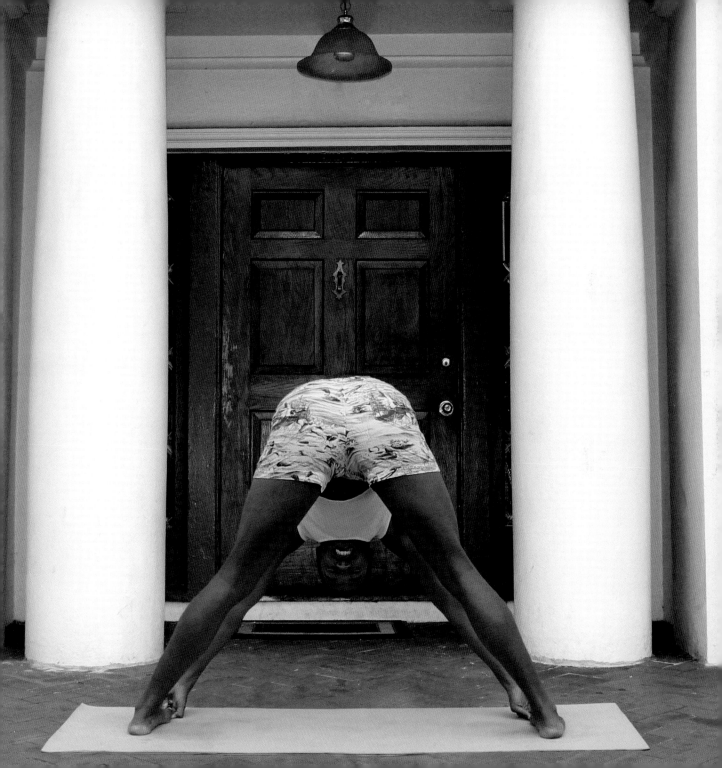

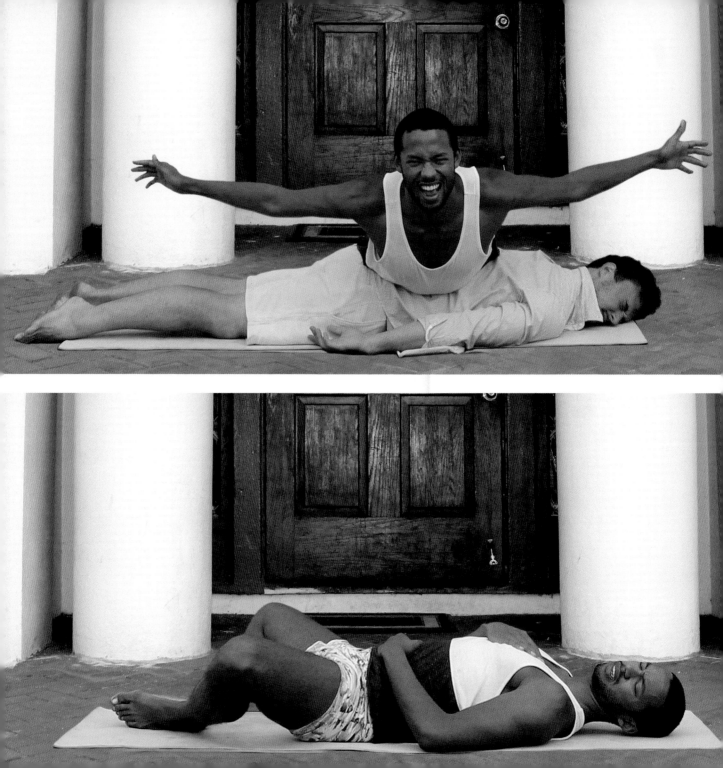

SUPERMAN TACKLEASANA

(OPPOSITE TOP)

Mindfully move in the direction of a nearby brogi. Breathe deeply and arch your back, then use a graceful tackle to flatten him like a pancake.

RECLINING BELLY ANGLE

(OPPOSITE BOTTOM)

After inhaling a large amount of chicken wings, lie down on your back. Let your knees fall out to the side to make way for your overextended belly. Bring the bottoms of your feet together and groan until your discomfort fades away.

MAKING YOGA FOR BROS
A LIFELONG PRACTICE

Congrats, brogi. You've reached the end of this book. But the end is only the beginning. You got a lot of fucking work to do.

For true brogis, life and practice are one. Each weight they curl or beer they touch becomes an opportunity to practice their brogic lifestyle. They do not distinguish between sticky mat and sticky, beer-soaked floor—both serve as an opportunity to breathe in and bro out.

So work the teachings of Yoga for Bros into all you do. And remember that Yoga for Bros is a package practice. You know what we mean . . . though each part of Yoga for Bros is beneficial, you must practice all parts to become the most badass of bros.

With the ways of Yoga for Bros to guide you, you'll learn how to one up our buddies, score more with the ladies, single-handedly support the American beer industry, rid yourself of the illness of emotions, and, with comfort-crushing commitment, reach true menlightenment.

ACKNOWLEDGMENTS

A big thanks to my models Trip, Sam, Hans, Kelly, Tim, Rob, Nick, Barron, David, Brian, and Jackson, the folks at Mission Cliffs and Triple Rock, my best proofreaders (that's you Mom and Dad!), Pim, Tess, and everyone else who made this book possible.

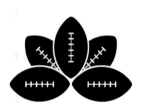

INDEX